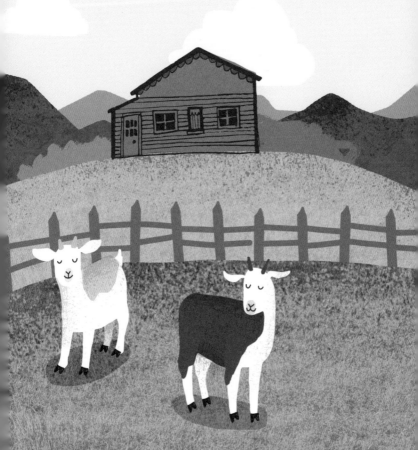

A BEGINNER'S GUIDE TO
GOAT YOGA

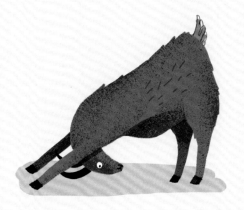

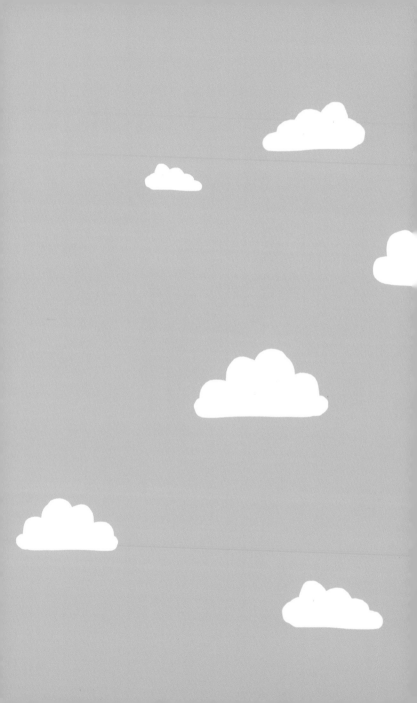

A BEGINNER'S GUIDE TO
GOAT YOGA
YES, IT IS ACTUALLY A THING

Sarah Jackson

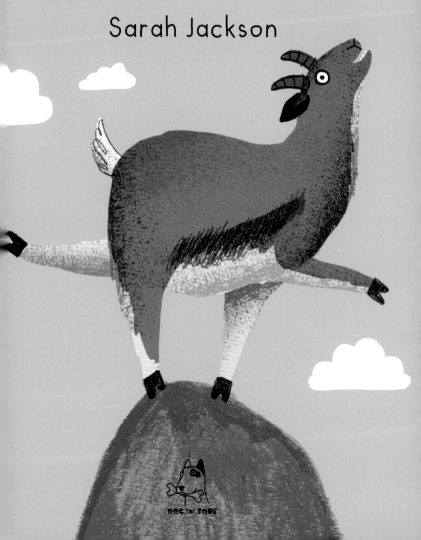

DOG 'n' BONE

Published in 2019 by Dog 'n' Bone Books
An imprint of Ryland Peters & Small Ltd
20-21 Jockey's Fields   341 E 116th St
London WC1R 4BW   New York, NY 10029

www.rylandpeters.com

10 9 8 7 6 5 4 3 2 1

Text © Sarah Jackson 2019
Design and illustration © Dog 'n' Bone Books 2019

A CIP catalog record for this book is available from the
Library of Congress and the British Library.

ISBN: 978 1 911026 85 3

Printed in China

Illustration and layout: Sarah Jackson

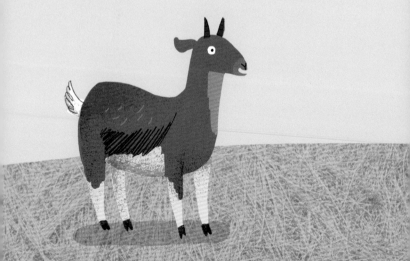

CONTENTS

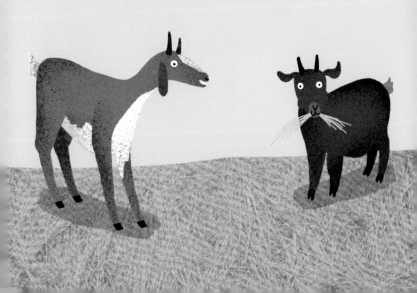

PART 1
WHAT IS GOAT YOGA?

Hello! I'm Gus.

I'm a Nigerian dwarf goat and somewhat of a goat yoga expert.

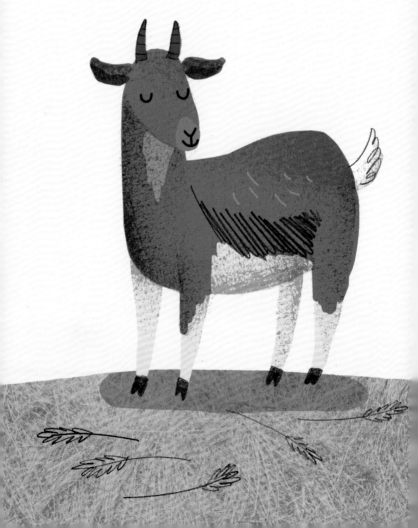

I'm here to talk about goat yoga, the new health phenomenon that's taking the world by storm. If you haven't heard of goat yoga, then I can only assume you've been hiding underground for the past year. Or that you are unfamiliar with this thing called the Internet.

This book will tell you all you need to know about goat yoga: what it is, how it came into being, why it's so great, and how you can start practicing, too.

So, let's get started... Firstly, what is goat yoga?

Well, of course, that's the first question I always get asked! Understandably so, as this concept is a relatively new one to a lot of people out there.

Since you're reading this book, I'm going to go with the following assumptions:

a) You do not know what goat yoga is.
b) Despite that, you are still a fairly intelligent person because you want to know what goat yoga is.
c) You can read*.

(*If you can't, don't worry too much because there are lots of pictures to help you along the way.)

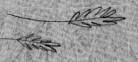

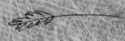

GREAT!

So, now that we've got that sorted, I'll begin.

Let's start with two basic definitions taken from the *Oxford English Dictionary*. I've highlighted the important bits:

YODEL
(verb)

A form of singing or calling marked by rapid alternation between the normal voice and falsetto.

Often accompanied by lederhosen—a strange sort of dungaree that should not be worn by anyone over 12 years old.

YOGA
(noun)

A Hindu spiritual discipline that is widely practiced for health and relaxation. It combines breath control, simple meditation, the adoption of specific bodily postures, and sometimes the practice of positivity mantras.

GOAT
(noun)

1. A hardy domesticated ruminant mammal that has backward-curving horns and (in the male) a beard. It is kept for its milk and meat, and noted for its lively behavior.

2. A lecherous man.

3. Informal: A stupid person; a fool.

GOATEE
(noun)
A small pointed beard like that of a goat. Popular among magicians and nineties' boy-band members.

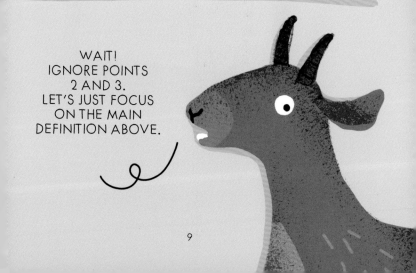

WAIT!
IGNORE POINTS
2 AND 3.
LET'S JUST FOCUS
ON THE MAIN
DEFINITION ABOVE.

So, if you put those two words together, what do you get? That's right... GOAT YOGA! Or as I like to call it: GOGA—a yoga workout, but with the addition of goats! It's the latest exercise to capture the imaginations and Instagram feeds of people all around the world. (Especially in America, of course!)

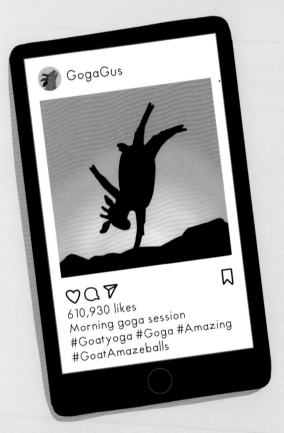

GogaGus

610,930 likes
Morning goga session
#Goatyoga #Goga #Amazing
#GoatAmazeballs

Goat yoga combines two of the best things ever. It's estimated over 20 million people around the world practice yoga. Of those that don't, many consider themselves to be "aspirational yogis" and wish that they did.

And goats? Well, we may not be quite so fashionable yet, but it's only a matter of time before everyone catches on to the fact that GOATS ARE BRILLIANT! If you are one of those people who doesn't know how great we are, then you soon will. Just look at this guy below. What's not to love?

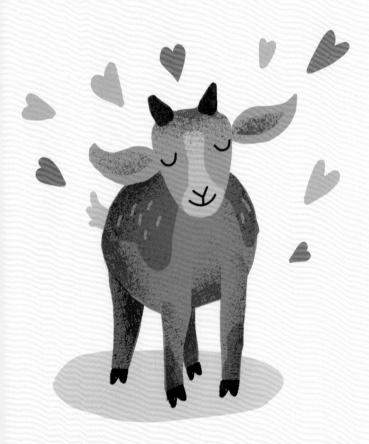

So, now that I've explained the million-dollar question, turn the page to take a look at how goat yoga began.

Although yoga has been practiced for thousands of years, the powers of goat yoga have only very recently been discovered.

The story starts on a small farm in Oregon, USA, set in rolling countryside and surrounded by beautiful mountains. The farm was owned by a very wise lady who knew how much fun it was to spend time with goats and the happiness and fulfillment they can bring to a person's life.

She would sometimes invite friends round to share the contentment that her goats would offer, and one day one of them made a great suggestion...

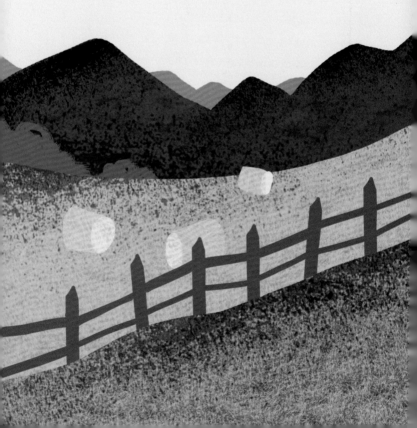

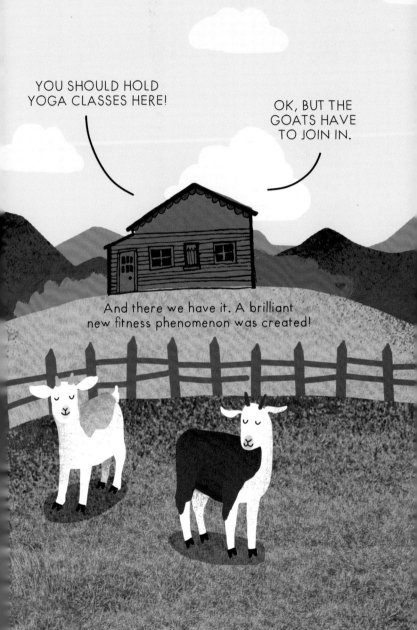

THE NEXT BIG THING

I know what you're thinking: "Not another fitness craze." Well, that couldn't be further from the truth. Sure, we've seen some rather strange fitness crazes over the last few decades...

HULA-HOOP

One of the biggest fitness fads of the 20th century, hula-hooping involves swinging a giant hoop repeatedly around one's tummy, apparently providing a fun way to tone your abs. Big in the '60s, not so much now.

PROS: Fun for 5 minutes.

CONS: Impossible for goats to use.

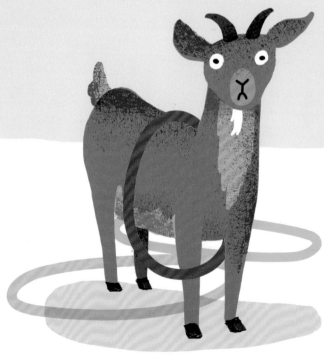

AIR SHORTS

Invented in the '70s, air shorts are one of the most bizarre fitness trends I've ever seen. These giant inflatable "exercise" shorts are designed to make you sweat away the pounds while going about your daily business.

PROS: Struggling to find any.

CONS: Make bathroom trips difficult. Prone to popping when you sit down. Make you sweat a lot. Look stupid.

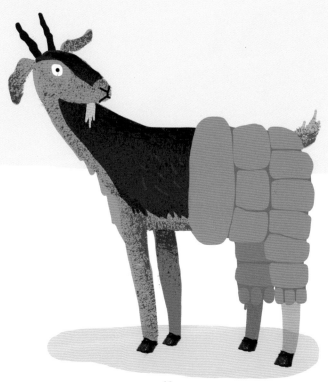

VIBRATION TECHNOLOGY

The likes of vibrating tummy belts and stand-on plates were big in the '90s and very popular among people with busy lives (or lazy folk). The idea is that small electronic pulses make your muscles move involuntarily, thus giving them a workout while you sit or stand around doing nothing.

PROS: You can watch TV and eat at the same time as "working out."

CONS: Feels weird. Not proven to work.

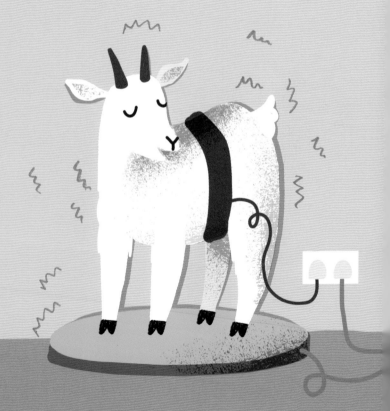

MERMAID SWIMMING

The newest sporting trend is mermaid swimming, which involves squeezing your back legs into a mermaid suit and diving through hoops.

PROS: Looks pretty.

CONS: Unsuitable for non-swimmers. And goats.

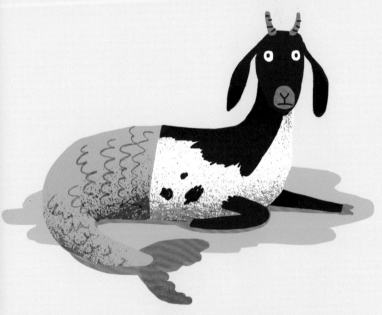

Thankfully, goat yoga's nothing like any of the above. For starters, both goats and yoga have been around for thousands of years and are still going strong! Plus, it's been scientifically proven that doing yoga or spending time with animals can improve your mood, health, and energy levels. I won't bore you with the science, but coming up are some of the amazing benefits of taking part in goat yoga...

GOAT YOGA BENEFITS

Taking part in regular yoga will help strengthen your muscles and joints, as well as increase your flexibility and posture. Goat yoga is about much more than that.

Practicing yoga surrounded by nature and a field of goats is exhilarating! It's not only good for your body, but it's great for your soul.

Those taking part can expect to see a big boost in their happy hormones. One happy Gogi compared goat yoga to drinking a bottle of wine, but without the double vision or hangover!

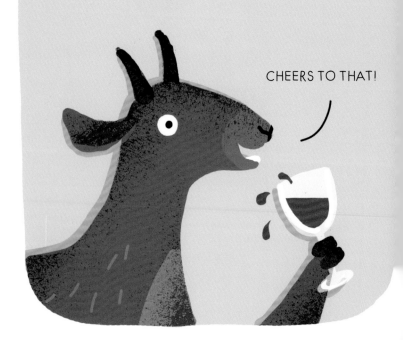

CHEERS TO THAT!

Wait, there's more: as your happy hormones increase, your stress levels will drop. Being around animals has been proven to reduce anxiety. Have you ever seen a stressed goat? No; that's because we are always in the company of other goats, so our stresses just slip away!

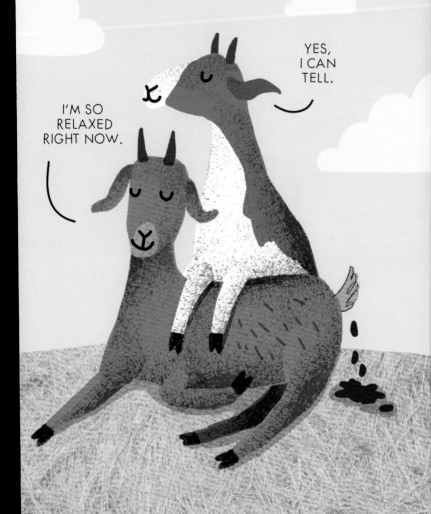

BUT WHY GOATS?

There's a common misconception going around that goats are just greedy and smelly. Well, frankly that's pretty offensive; there is way more to us than that.

Did you know that goats were one of the first animals to be tamed by humans over 9,000 years ago? Look back through the history books and you'll find many a cave painting of the trusty goat.

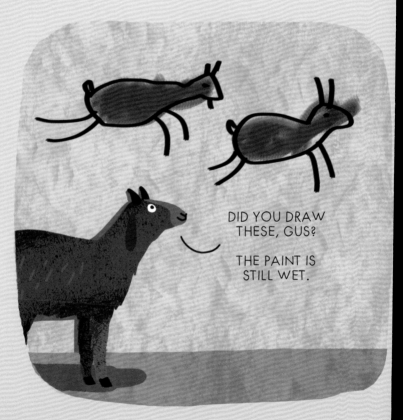

DID YOU DRAW THESE, GUS?

THE PAINT IS STILL WET.

Although we are great for farming, we're also a very sociable lot who love to spend time in the company of other goats and humans.

People often hail the dog as man's best friend, but I've got some news for you! Recent scientific research shows that goats are just as intelligent as dogs AND can outlive them by a few years. Plus, as well as making fantastic companions we can also provide help with household chores, like keeping the garden lawn trim.

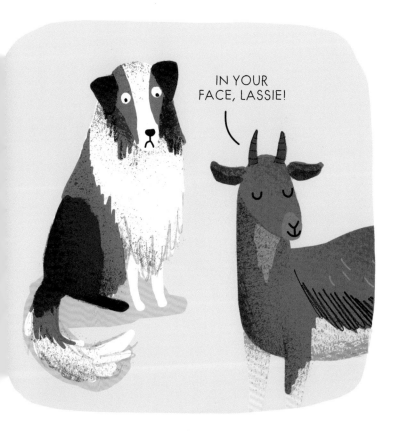

IN YOUR FACE, LASSIE!

Goats have achieved some amazing things that may have gone under the radar. We've held some pretty important positions in our time and have helped shape history.

CULTURAL IMPACT

Did you know that goats discovered the stimulating effects of coffee? That's right! Goat farmers in the Middle Ages noticed their animals dancing and acting "excitably" after eating coffee berries, so you can thank my ancestors for your morning espresso hit!

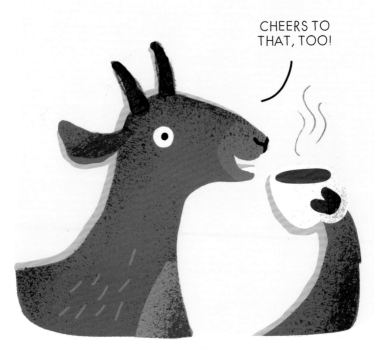

CHEERS TO THAT, TOO!

POLITICAL STATUS

In 1986, Clay Henry, the "beer-drinking goat," was elected Mayor of Lajitas, Texas. He became the town's most popular tourist attraction and even starred in some movies. He was so successful as Mayor that he has been followed by many goat successors. Clay Moore Henry was elected in 2014 and currently is doing a great job.

IT'S A TOUGH JOB, BUT SOMEONE'S GOTTA DO IT. *HICCUP*

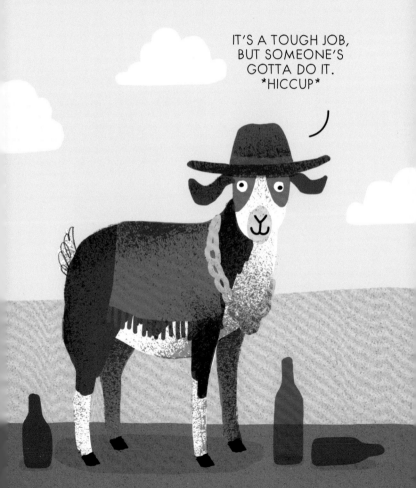

MILITARY HISTORY

Did you know that goats have served in the military since 1775, and have even accompanied troops on the battlefields? One of the most renowned military goats was Lance Corporal William Windsor, who served in the British Army from 2001 until 2009. He hit the headlines after being demoted for inappropriate behavior during the Queen's birthday party, where he tried to head-butt a drummer. He was reinstated after animal rights groups campaigned on his behalf. They knew he was just kidding around.

WHO KNEW THOSE ROYALS TOOK THINGS SO SERIOUSLY?

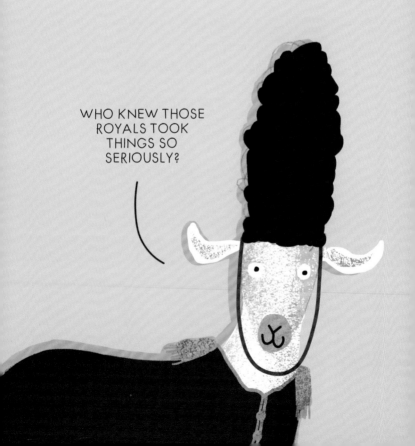

SPORTING ACHIEVEMENTS

We love taking part in active pursuits and can even boast some world records. In 2013, Happie, a goat from Florida, broke the Guinness World Record for the farthest distance traveled by a goat on a skateboard, covering 120 feet in 25 seconds.

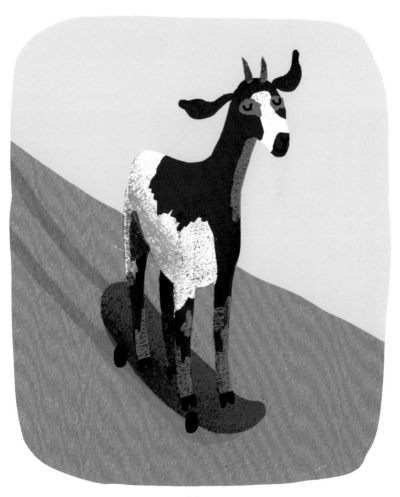

Anyway, I don't think you need any more convincing about how great we goats are. Instead, let's get back to talking about why yoga and goats are a match made in heaven.

You've probably thought about trying yoga with some other animals too, like your trusty pet dog. Well, let me stop you right there. We put some other animals to the test and the results just weren't good...

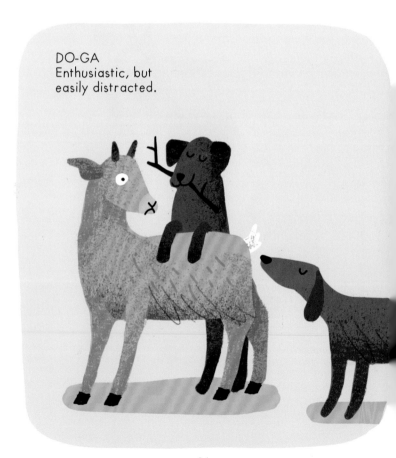

DO-GA
Enthusiastic, but
easily distracted.

CAT-GA
Very flexible, but they're lazy and have poor interaction skills.

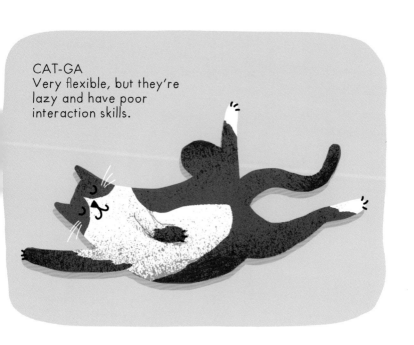

TORTOI-GA
Good at meditating, but don't expect much of a workout.

YOU OK, NIGEL? YOU HAVEN'T MOVED FOR THREE WEEKS.

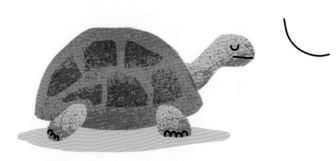

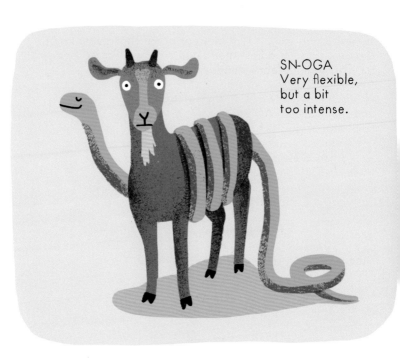

SN-OGA
Very flexible,
but a bit
too intense.

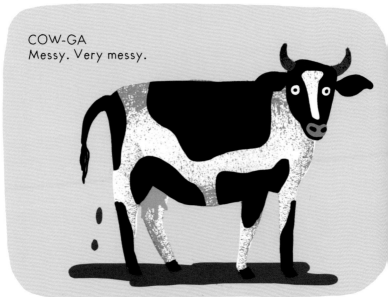

COW-GA
Messy. Very messy.

So there you have it. If that's not proof that goats make the best yoga buddies, then I don't know what else can be. Oh, wait, celebrity endorsements!

Those famous folk are always first to spot a good thing, and there are LOADS who have enjoyed yoga in the company of goats. From '70s rock stars on family vacations to A-list celebrities at their birthday parties, we've heard of countless VIPs who love a spot of goat yoga. Of course, I can't mention any names, because those star types insist on maintaining their privacy, but I can assure you they all had a great time.

Hopefully one of them will put me in touch with a hot-shot director, so that I can star in my own fitness video and become famous myself one day...

That's my Hollywood star.

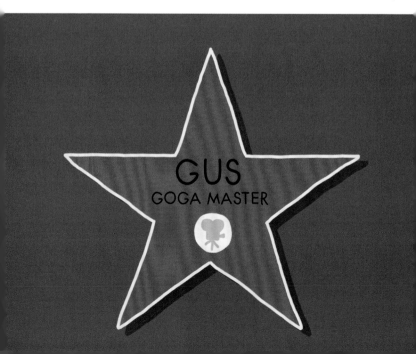

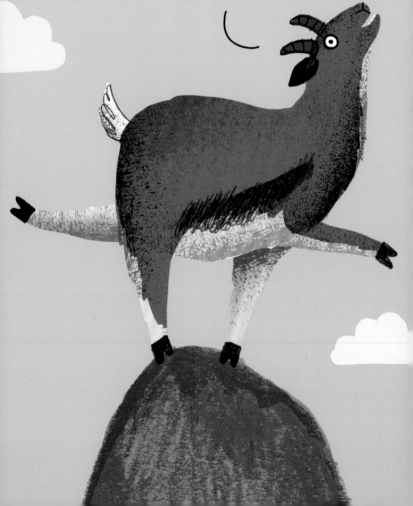

CONVINCED? OK, LET'S TAKE YOU THROUGH SOME BASIC POSES...

PART 2
GOAT YOGA POSITIONS

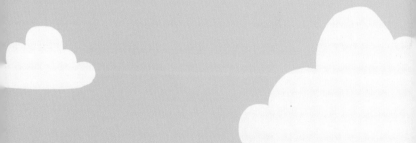

DOWNWARD-FACING GOAT

Yoga's most infamous pose! This one's great for a deep back- and leg-stretch. It's perfect for blowing away the cobwebs after a long day of grazing the paddock, or whatever you humans do all day.

PLEASE NOTE: This pose is known for triggering the passing of wind. So if you are near a spider's web, please be careful you don't literally blow those cobwebs away.

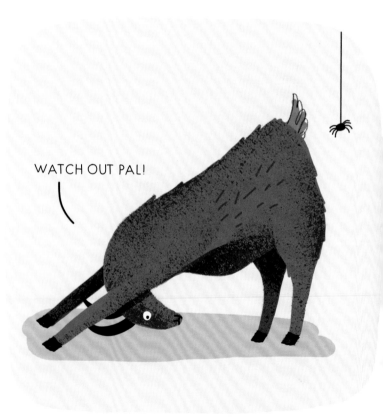

THE PLANK

This is an arm-balancing yoga pose that tones the abdominal muscles while strengthening the arms and spine. We goats aren't built like you human-folk and have had to make a few adaptations. But please be reassured that, whatever it looks like, we are definitely giving it 100% and are not just taking a snack break.

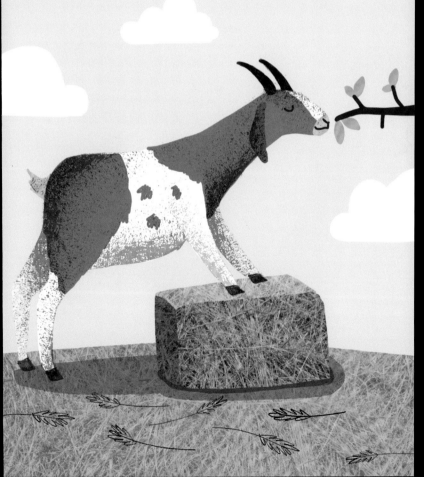

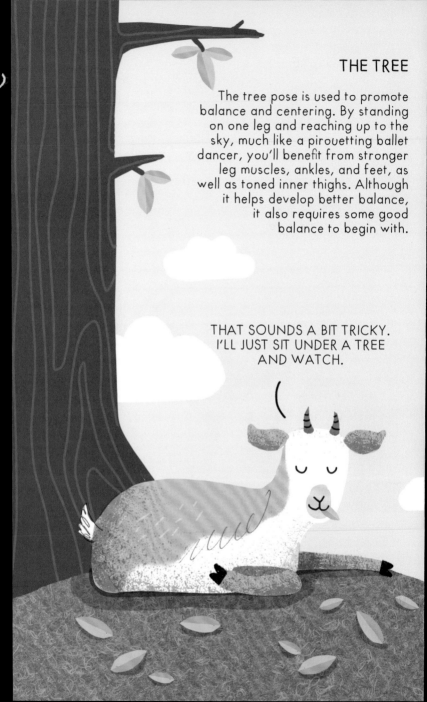

THE TREE

The tree pose is used to promote balance and centering. By standing on one leg and reaching up to the sky, much like a pirouetting ballet dancer, you'll benefit from stronger leg muscles, ankles, and feet, as well as toned inner thighs. Although it helps develop better balance, it also requires some good balance to begin with.

THAT SOUNDS A BIT TRICKY. I'LL JUST SIT UNDER A TREE AND WATCH.

WARRIOR POSE

The traditional warrior pose is a little like the lunge position. It's meant to symbolize spiritual strength and the courage to face your foes. We goats have developed our own version of this pose that's a lot more fun. We like to lock horns and wrestle!

You may think this looks a bit aggressive, or that we're not getting along with each other, but that's not true. It's our way of playing and bonding with one another. Don't be surprised if you receive a gentle nudge from one of us while performing your downward goat. It just means we like you.

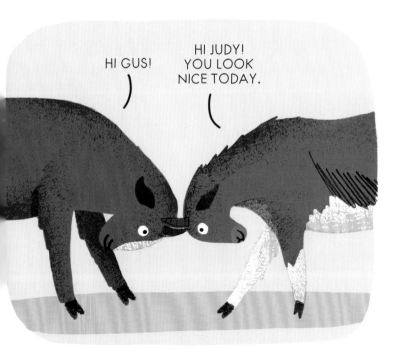

HAPPY BABY POSE

The happy baby pose is a brilliant one for releasing your inner kid. It's easy for beginners and it's a great mood booster. The pose itself is very simple to master and is ideal for a hip stretch. However, us goats do sometimes struggle to get back up again and may require a little push to help us along the way.

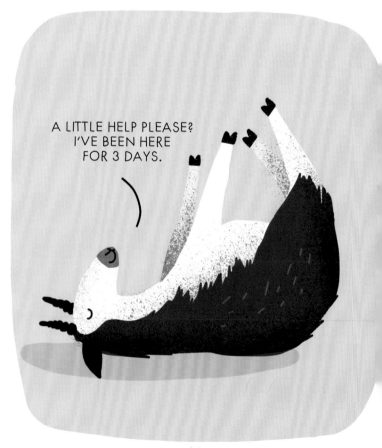

MOUNTAIN POSE

The mountain pose, known as Tadasana to us experts, is a super pose. To the untrained eye, it may look like you are just standing still, but, when done properly, you will use every muscle in your body.

This pose will strengthen your back, tummy, thighs, knees, ankles, and, most importantly, your buttocks. Just look at that rump!

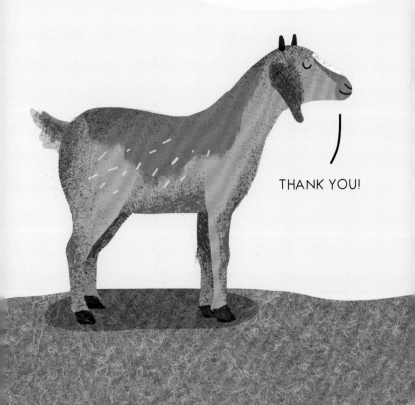

THANK YOU!

This herd of mountain goats are masters of their art. It may look to you like they are asleep, but they are in fact just really focused on their mountain poses and their third eyes*.

*"THIRD EYE" DEFINITION:
Gateway to higher consciousness and symbol of enlightenment, which is often sought after in ancient yoga meditation practices. Also known as the "inner eye." Not to be confused with an actual third eye.

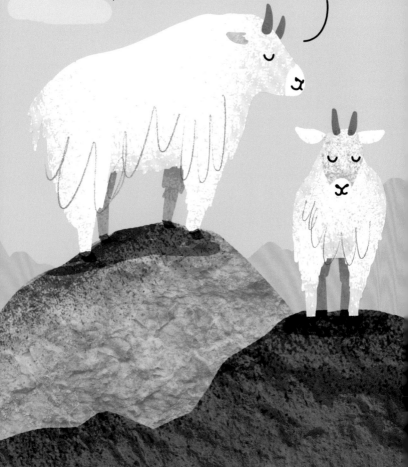

I SPY WITH MY THIRD EYE...

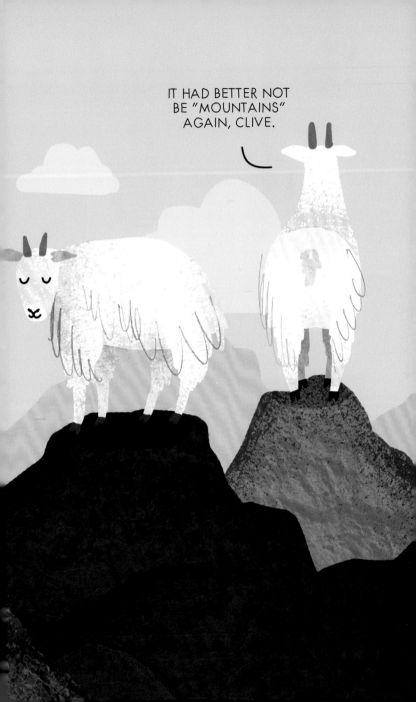

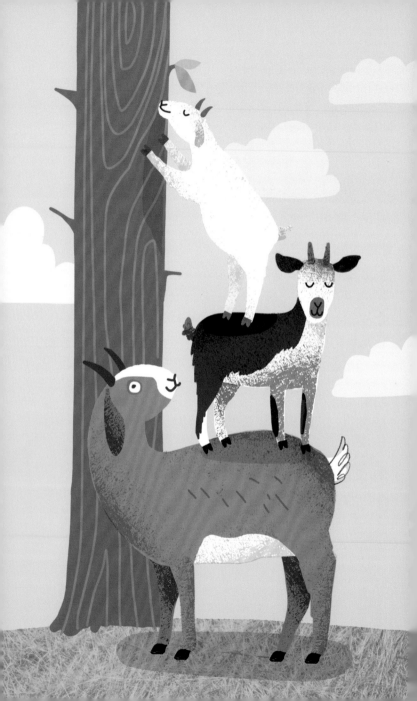

PYRAMID POSE

The pyramid pose is a standing yoga posture that combines the benefits of three major movements: forward bending, backward bending, and balancing. It requires a lot of focus and a very calm mind to keep your balance and stay in the correct position.

We've adapted our own version of the pyramid pose, which is equally challenging but a whole lot more fun. You'll need some buddies for this one—and that's where we come in! Added benefits of the goga pyramid pose include a free back massage for the bottom and middle tiers, and a great view (plus some potential snacking opportunities) for the top member of the pyramid team!

We'd advise you humans to stick to the bottom tier, because you're not natural climbers like us.

ROOM FOR A LITTLE ONE?

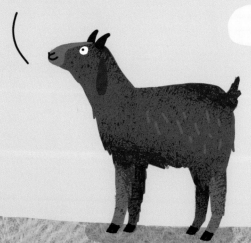

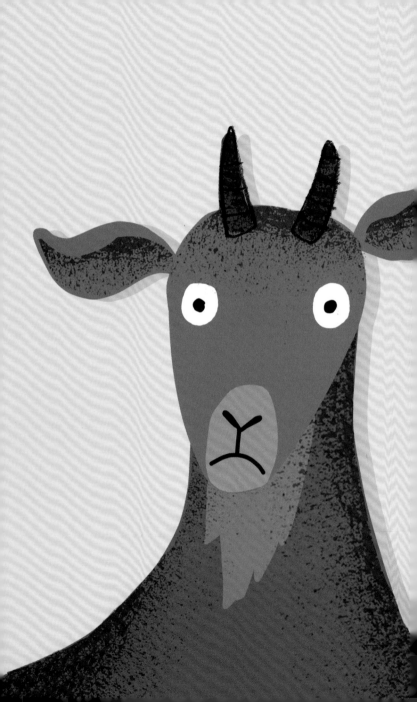

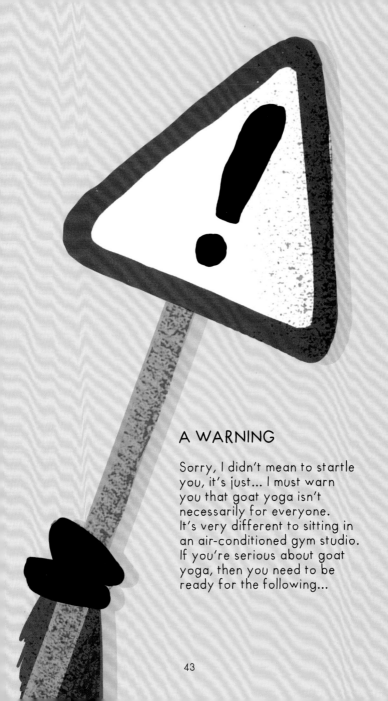

A WARNING

Sorry, I didn't mean to startle you, it's just... I must warn you that goat yoga isn't necessarily for everyone. It's very different to sitting in an air-conditioned gym studio. If you're serious about goat yoga, then you need to be ready for the following...

43

1. WE PRACTICE OUTDOORS

This allows us goats to feel relaxed in our natural environment, while allowing you to enjoy the nature and some lovely fresh air. Forget polished floors and wall-to-wall mirrors; you will be practicing on grass, surrounded by hay bales (which are tasty, but sometimes a bit itchy if the hay gets in the wrong places). As such, you'll need to be prepared to face the elements from time to time. That's right... Wind and rain. I'd recommend wearing a good waterproof trench coat or poncho--both sensible and stylish.

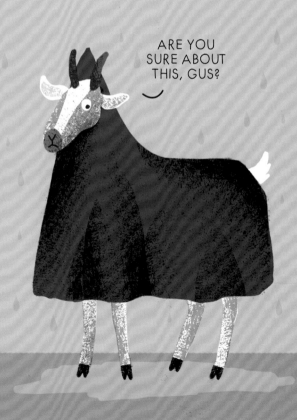

ARE YOU
SURE ABOUT
THIS, GUS?

Sometimes, it can be quite hot and sunny (although probably not if you live in the UK), so just remember that the only air-con you'll have is nature's wind on your face. If you're unlucky, you may have some goat's wind in your face, too. Make sure you apply a liberal layer of sunscreen before taking part in your yoga session. You want to be able to focus on your downward-goat pose without worrying about burning your booty. I like to wear some shades and a visor, along with a good dollop of sunblock. That way I'm not only fully protected, but also look super cool.

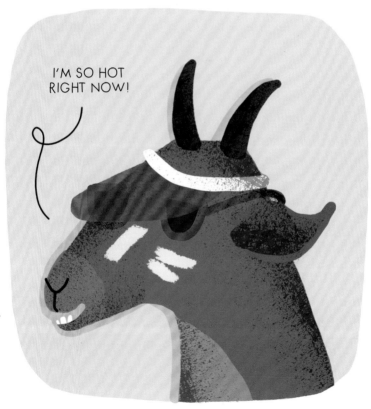

I'M SO HOT RIGHT NOW!

2. GOATS LIKE EATING

I'm not just talking about grass and hay here. We goats enjoy a varied diet and are known to be experimental when it comes to dining. I would advise that you don't come to goat yoga in your latest fancy fitness clothes, unless you don't mind a few extra "ventilation holes" being created. We take regular snack breaks throughout the day and can't be held responsible for what may end up in our stomachs.

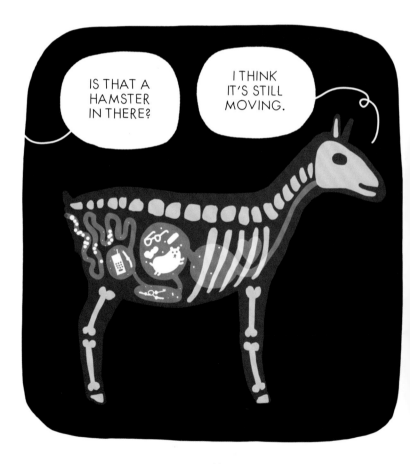

You may be asked to sign a waiver to make sure you understand the extent of our appetites. It will probably look something like this:

WARNING!

OUR GOATS CANNOT BE HELD RESPONSIBLE FOR WHAT THEY EAT. ANY LOSS OR DAMAGE OF PERSONAL POSSESSIONS WILL BE AT THE OWNER'S RISK.

This includes, but is not limited to the following:

Grass lawns
Fences
Yoga mats
Loose clothing
Fitted clothing
Underwear
Jewelry
Hair

Wigs
Hipster beards
Non-hipster beards
Purses/wallets
Money (both notes and coins)
Bus tickets
Passports
Pocket fluff

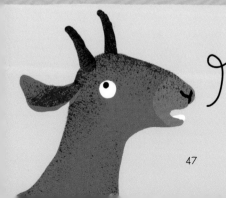

BORING ALERT!

JUST SIGN YOUR NAME ON THE LINE AND LET'S GET DOWN TO THE FUN STUFF.

3. GOATS ARE FLATULENT

Yes, I suppose it's about time we got to this bit. Goats are very windy animals, with four stomachs to help digest our varied diet of food. That intensive fermentation process, when combined with certain yoga positions, tends to result in rather a lot of excess gas.

Don't be surprised if you hear the odd burp or parp coming from a nearby goat—it's really very normal. And, besides, you can always blame a goat if you accidentally make your own yoga-parp!

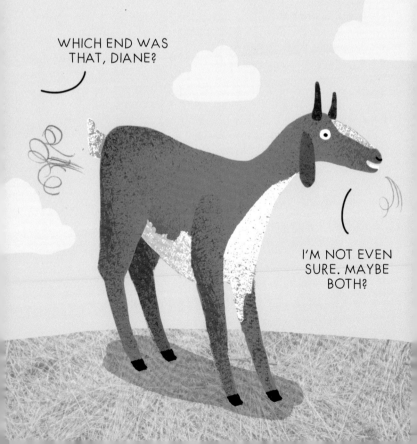

4. GOATS DON'T USE A TOILET

Sorry to break it to you, but we aren't potty trained, and we don't like wearing diapers. We will go when the mood takes us, which may be during your yoga class. Here are a couple of things you should look out for when taking part in goat yoga:

Anything that resembles chocolate. It may be a chocolate-covered raisin, but it probably isn't.

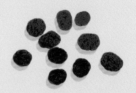

Yellow puddles.

The goat who's been eating non-stop all through your class. It's only a matter of time.

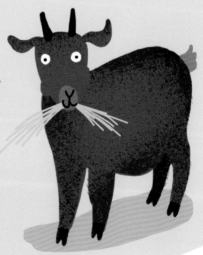

WHAT MAKES A GOOD GOGI?

It's not easy to reach and maintain Gogi status. It takes regular practice and training to be the best! Here's how I stay on top of my game:

POSITIVITY

A gloomy goat makes for a poor yoga companion. I practice smiling daily to make sure I radiate good vibes.

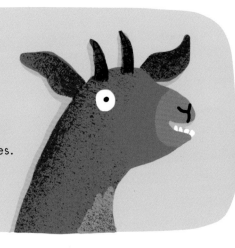

INTELLIGENCE AND MINDFULNESS

I keep my mind sharp by reading one book a week. Sometimes I read non-fiction, but I do love a good detective novel!

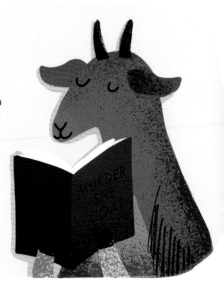

FLEXIBILITY AND BALANCE

I try to find ways of incorporating stretching and balancing into my everyday tasks to get as much practice as possible.

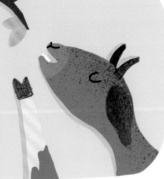

GOOD PERSONAL HYGIENE

Before each class, I like to freshen up by rolling around in the nearest available shrub to ensure I always come out smelling delectable. My faves are lavender and rosemary. Watch out for those stinging nettles though...

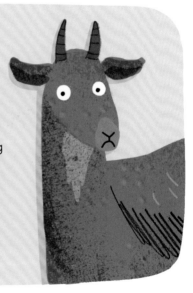

There you have it, my guide to being a great Gogi! It takes a lot of practice and hard work, but you do also need to be blessed with the right physical and character attributes. Overleaf are some of the goats that didn't quite make the grade...

HAIRY GOATS

Risk of overheating. Excess molting is unpleasant to be around. Obscured vision can be dangerous.

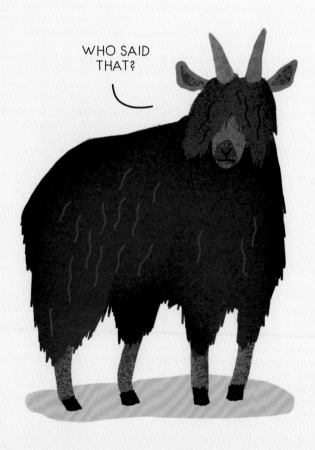

LONG-HORNED GOATS

Just dangerous.

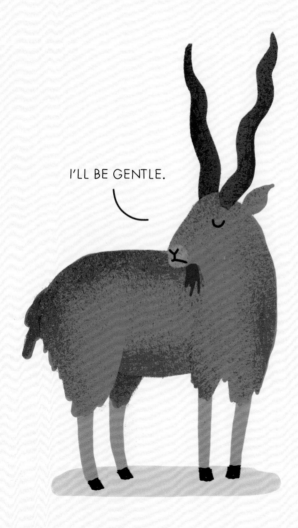

I'LL BE GENTLE.

SHEEP MASQUERADING AS GOATS

Don't let the horns and fur confuse you. Sheep are far too stupid to master the art of yoga.

BUT I LOVE YODA.

IT'S YO-GA

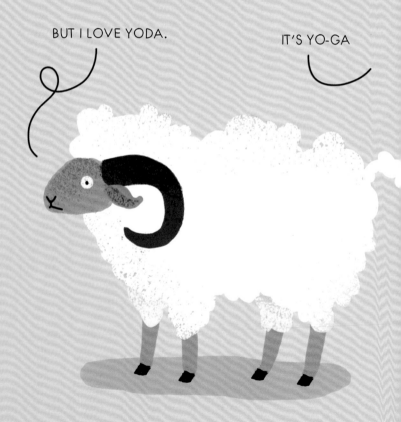

FAINTING GOATS

We recently introduced a ban on myotonic goats, otherwise known as fainting goats, who have been known to pass out when startled. At first we thought yoga might help them relax, but it became difficult to work out if they were in a yoga pose or had just passed out.

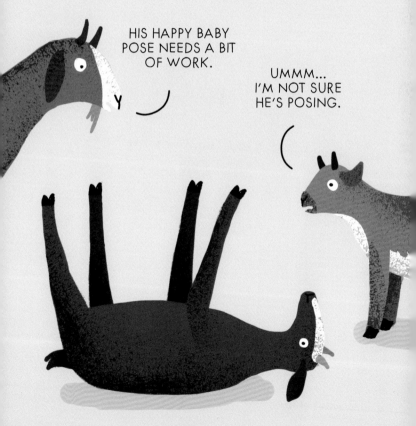

Obviously, I can't teach goat yoga everywhere, but that's OK! There are lots of fantastic goga teachers all over the world that are spreading the good word and sharing their goat wisdom with you lucky humans...

Like my cousin John O'Goat in Scotland.

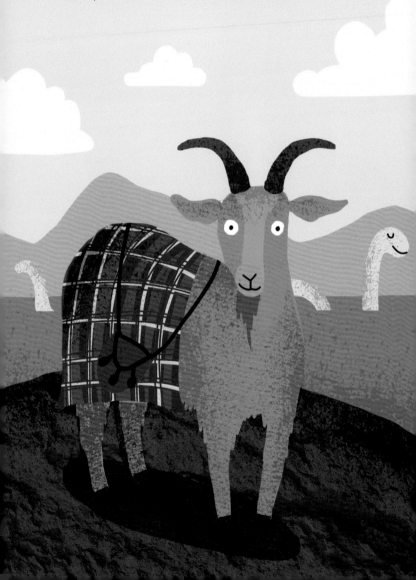

And one of the oldest and wisest Gogis out there, the Goatfather. He's one of the original founders of the goat yoga movement. No one knows how old he is, but there are rumors floating about that say he has fathered thousands of goats. It's true that he commands the utmost respect, but he's not to be confused with the Godfather from the movies (he hates that).

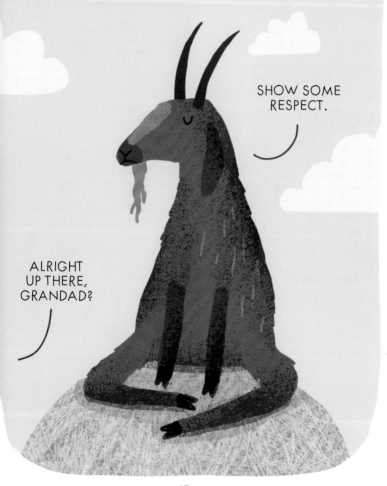

SHOW SOME RESPECT.

ALRIGHT UP THERE, GRANDAD?

Goat yoga has changed the lives of many people, bringing them joy, peace, fun, relaxation, calmness, happiness, and a release from the things in life that can get you down. We've had hundreds of letters from people telling us how much goat yoga means to them and how it has enriched their lives, but it's not just you humans who love it. Here's what some of my goat pals have to say...

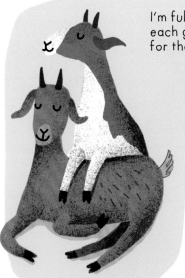

I'm full of happy hormones after each goga class and can't wait for the next one!

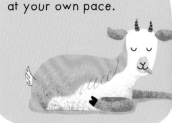

It's challenging and fun, but you can go at your own pace.

Goga is so welcoming and friendly—for goats of all shapes and sizes. I've made some great friends who accept me for who I am.

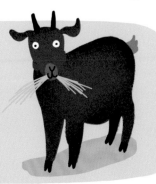

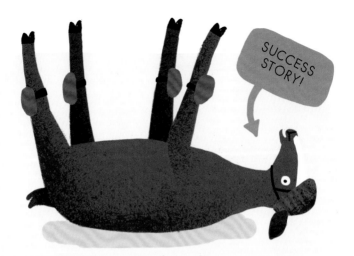

I definitely feel more relaxed since starting goga. I still suffer with my nerves, but it's improving each day. Gus suggested I wear protective clothing for the fainting, so I can keep coming to classes now; which is great!

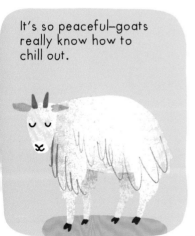

It's so peaceful—goats really know how to chill out.

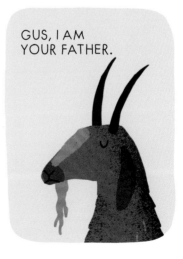

GUS, I AM YOUR FATHER.

CONGRATULATIONS!

You're now familiar with goat yoga! All that's left to do is for you to take the plunge and find your nearest goga school. Now that you're prepared for all of the eventualities, there really is nothing to stop you.

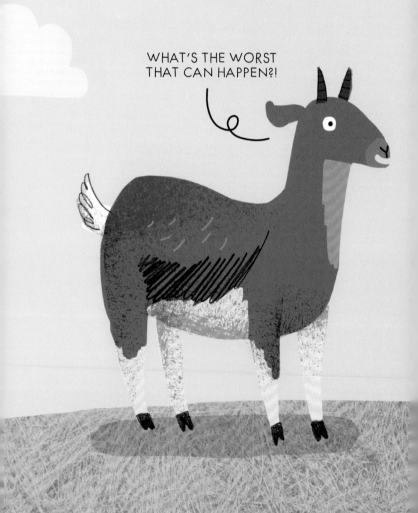

WHAT'S THE WORST THAT CAN HAPPEN?!

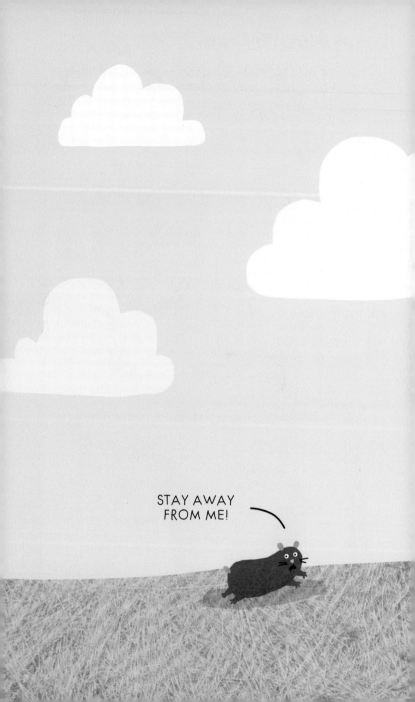

GOAT HALL OF FAME

Just in case this book hasn't done enough to convince you how great we truly are, I'll leave you with some of our most famous goats to remind you one more time...

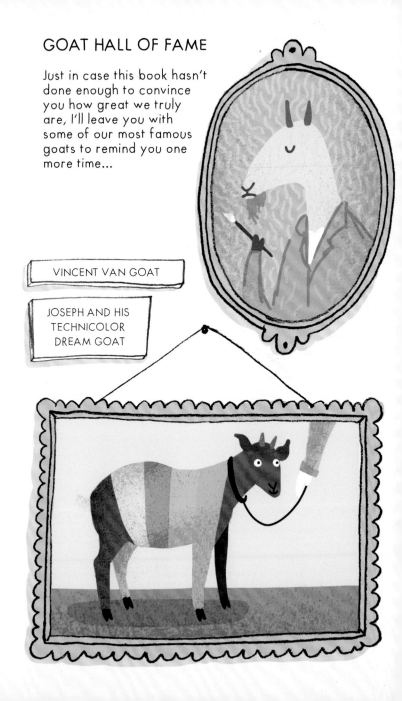

VINCENT VAN GOAT

JOSEPH AND HIS TECHNICOLOR DREAM GOAT

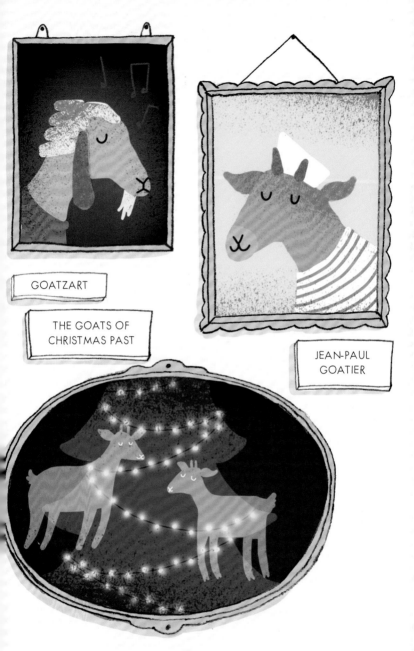

GOATZART

THE GOATS OF
CHRISTMAS PAST

JEAN-PAUL
GOATIER

Acknowledgments

I'd like to dedicate this book to my wonderful group of friends, who are always happy to help brainstorm goat puns at the pub, and are the first to tell me when my goats "look a bit weird."

Namaste.

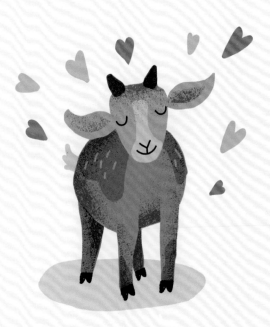

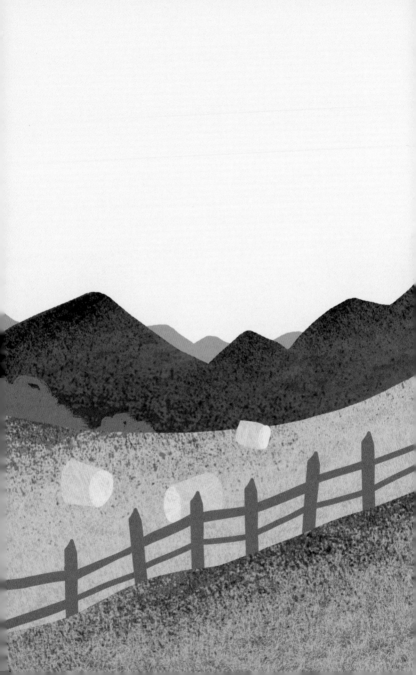